# Titus' Adventure Guidebook

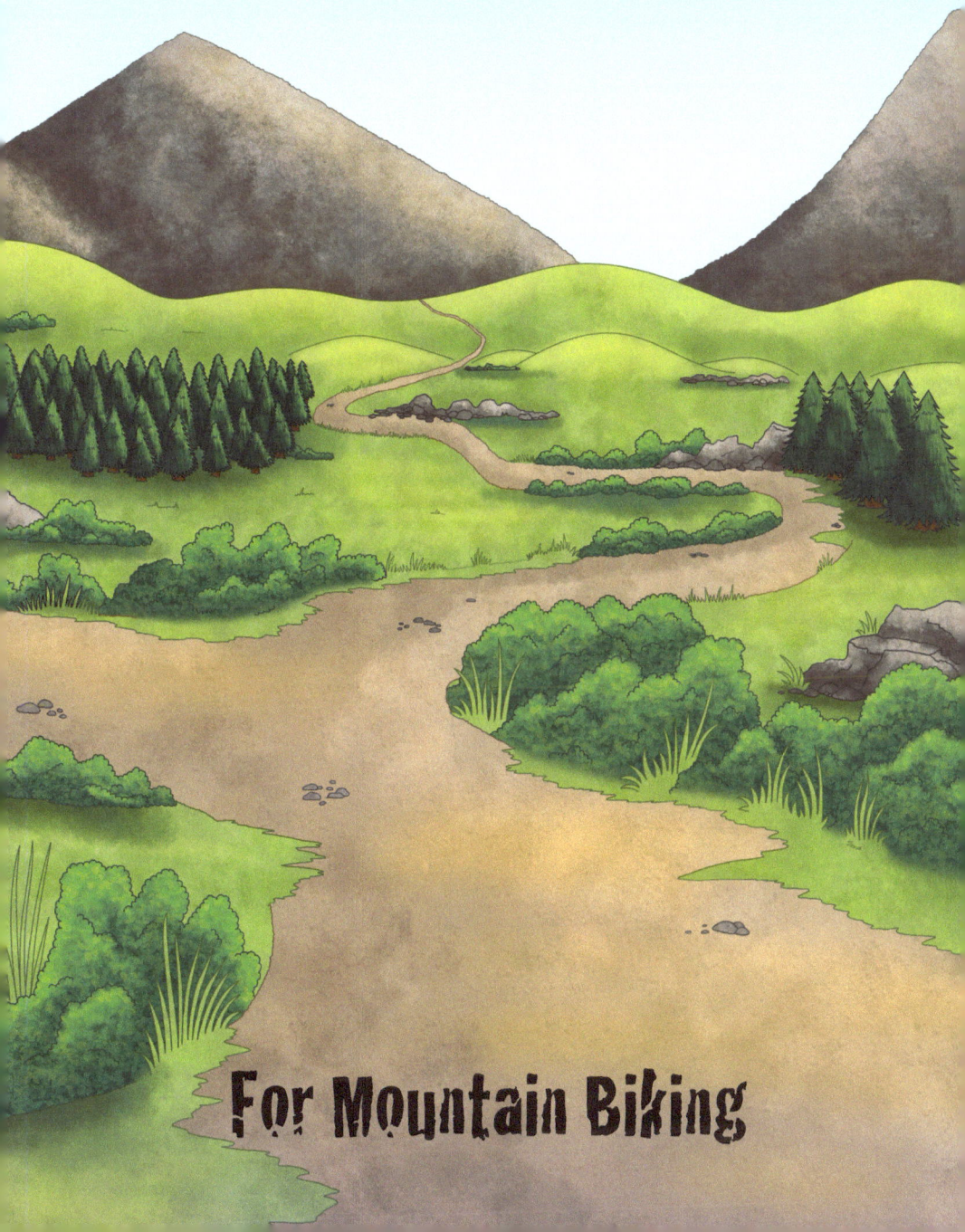

# For Mountain Biking

1st book in the TAG SERIES
Titus' Adventure Guidebook For Mountain Biking
copyright © 2010 by Coach Cathleen. Illustrations
copyright © 2013 by Lauren Scott. All rights
reserved. Produced and distributed in the USA,
2013 by CC Training LLC.

ISBN: 978-0-9898050-0-1
Library of Congress Control Number: 2013914177

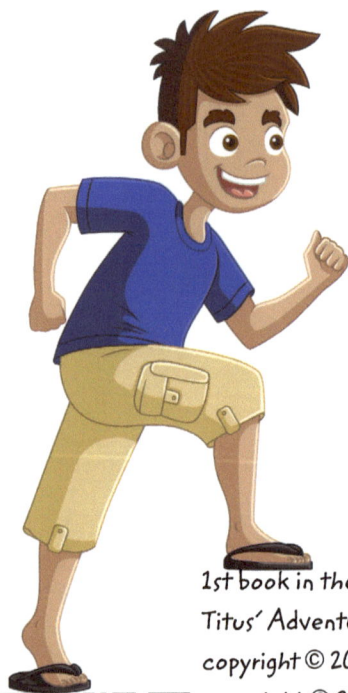

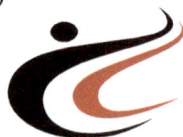

Scan with RedLaser

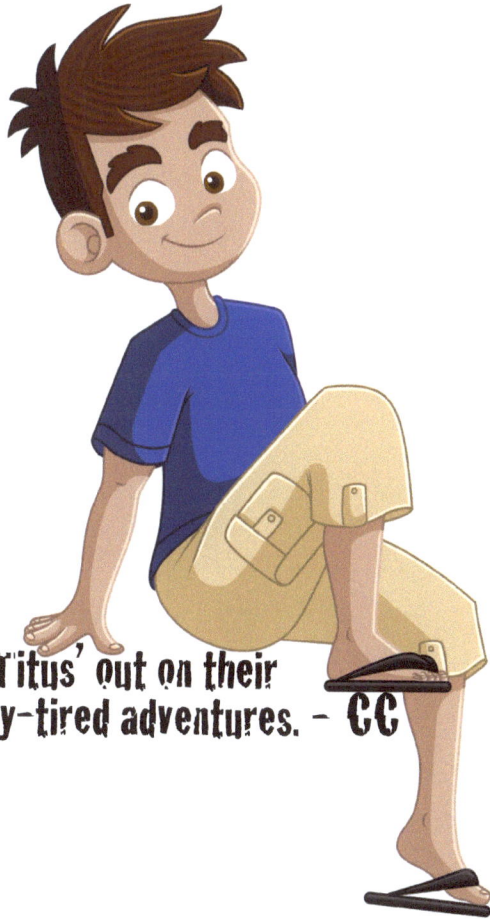

To all the Titus' out on their
knobby-tired adventures. - CC

Oh hi, my name is Titus. I'm getting ready to go on a mountain bike ride!

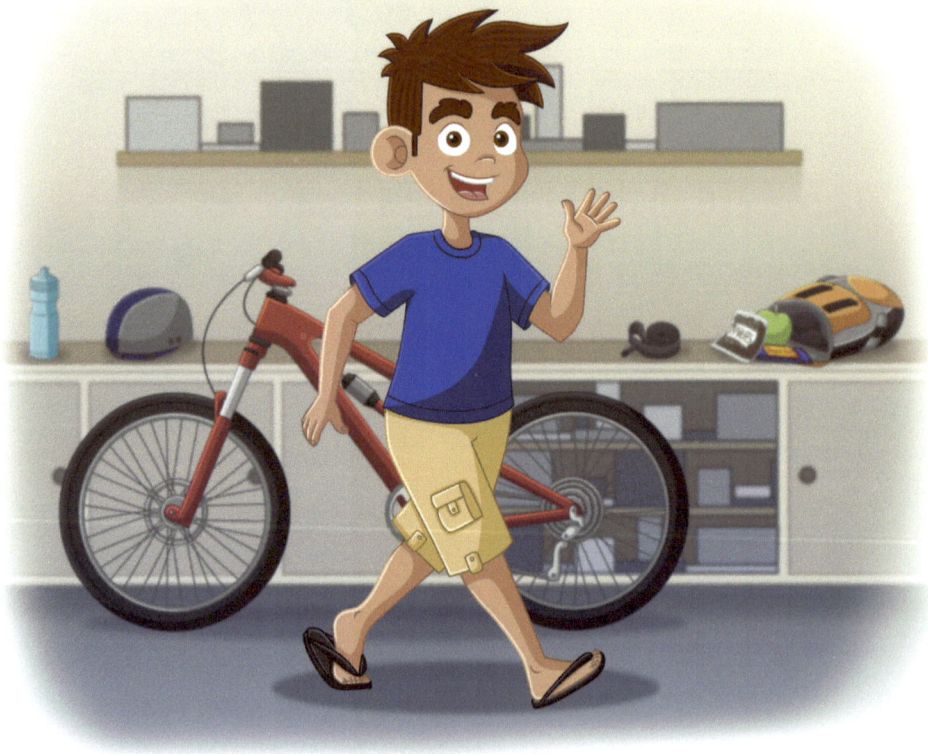

I can hardly wait to be up in the hills on my mountain bike!

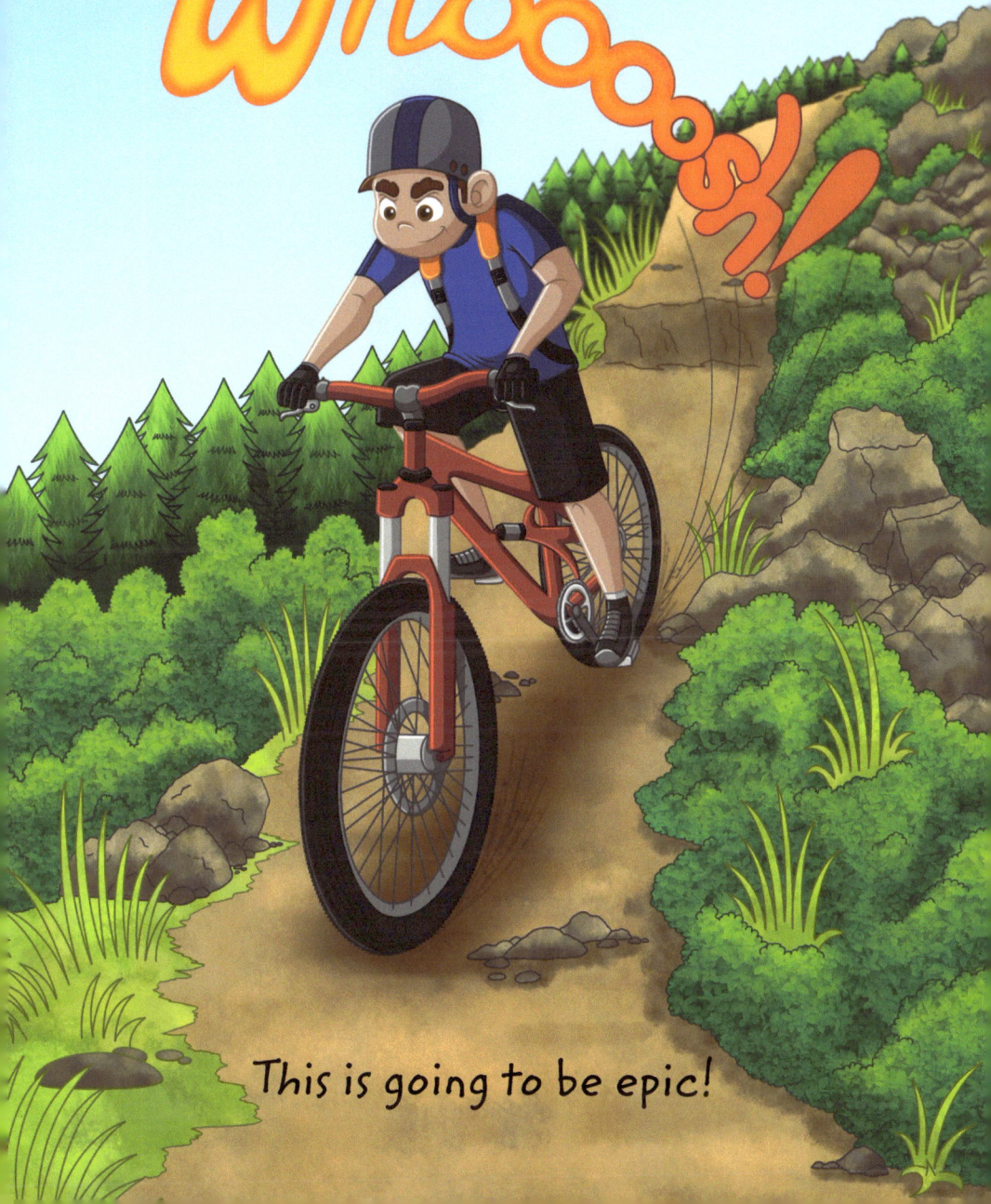

Bombing down the dirt trail, my knobby tires buzzing below me, catchin' air and the fresh wind in my face.

Whoooosh!

This is going to be epic!

There are a few things to get ready before my ride.

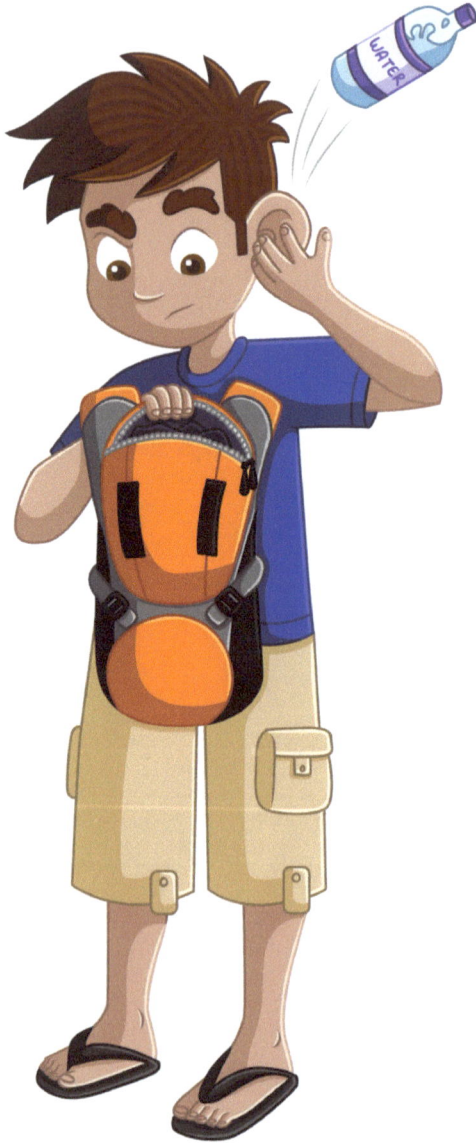

I will need to get all of my gear together.

I always wear my bike helmet when I ride —
Mom says it will keep my noggin from getting
misshapen if I accidentally <u>go over the falls</u>- I
think it helps keep the sun off my face.

Mountain Bike

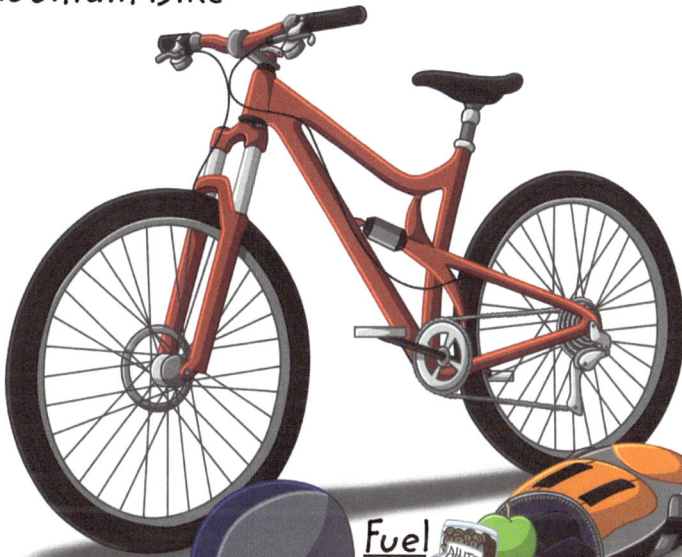

<u>Fuel</u>

Helmet

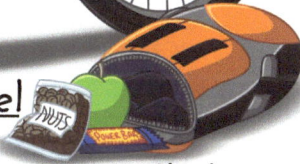

Hydration Pack/
Water Bottle

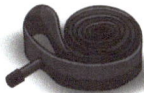

Spare Tube

Wow, that looks like a lot of stuff! Sometimes I
even need a compact bike pump, tire levers, and
patch kit but today my motley-mountain-biking
crew is sharing the load.

# Alright

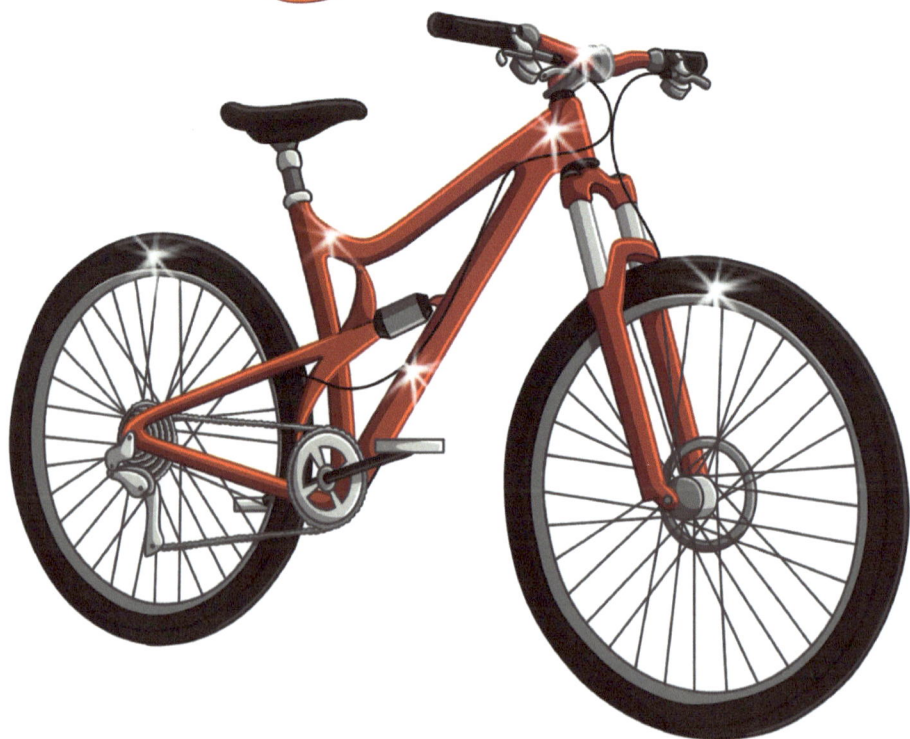

My buddy checked over my bike and chain
to make sure it was all working well!

It sure is nice riding with other people so we can all help each other along the way. Aside from being safer, it's neat to watch my friends have fun on their bikes too!

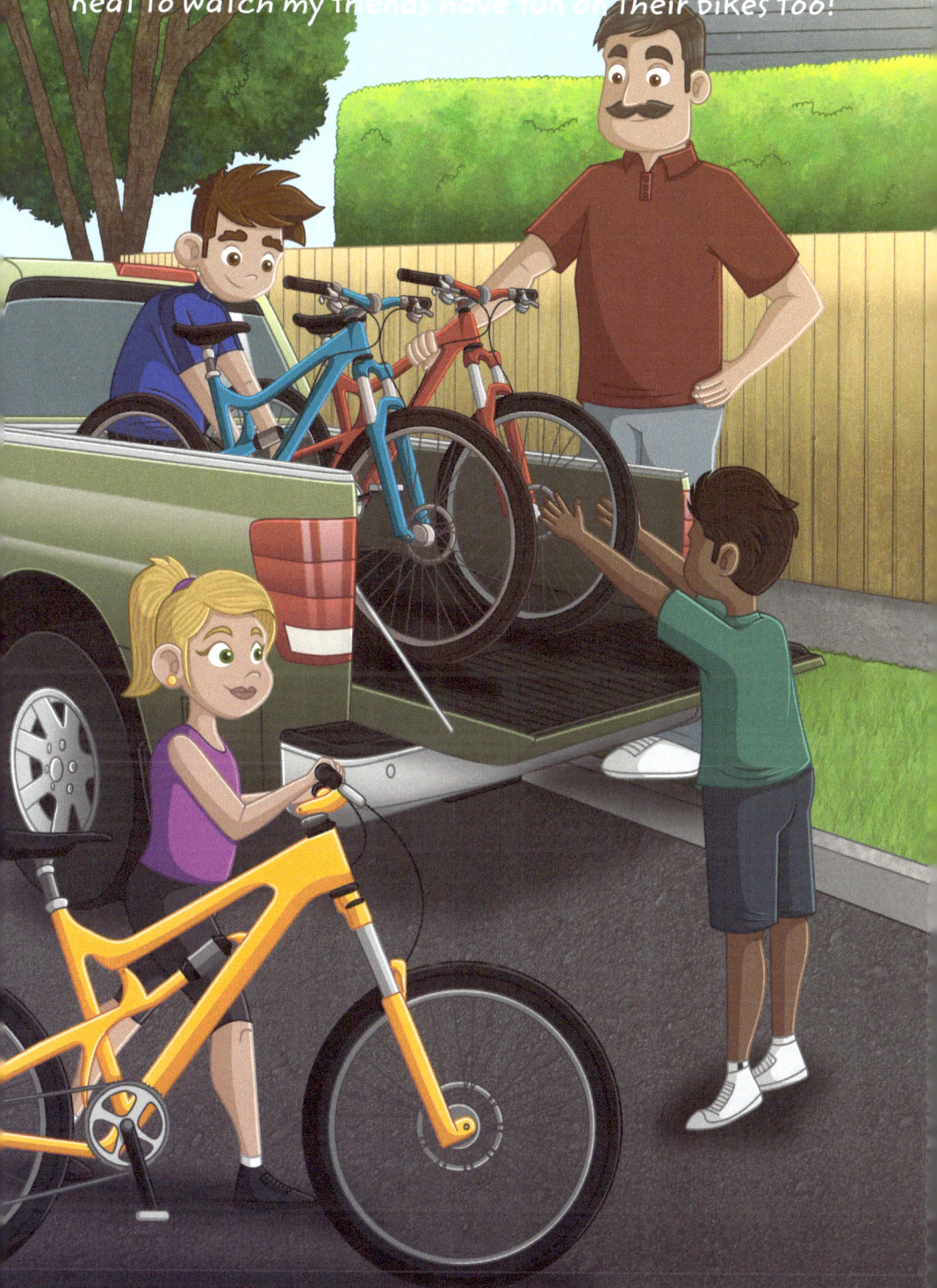

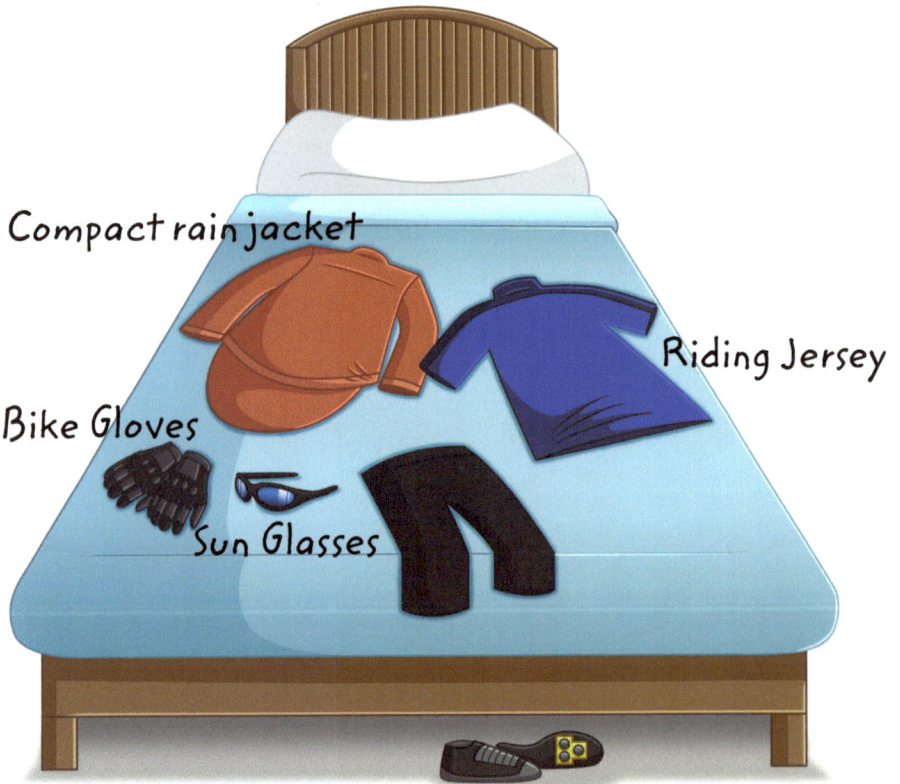

Now then, what to wear?

Compact rain jacket

Riding Jersey

Bike Gloves

Sun Glasses

I like wearing my sunglasses because they protect my eyes.
Plus I think they look pretty cool.

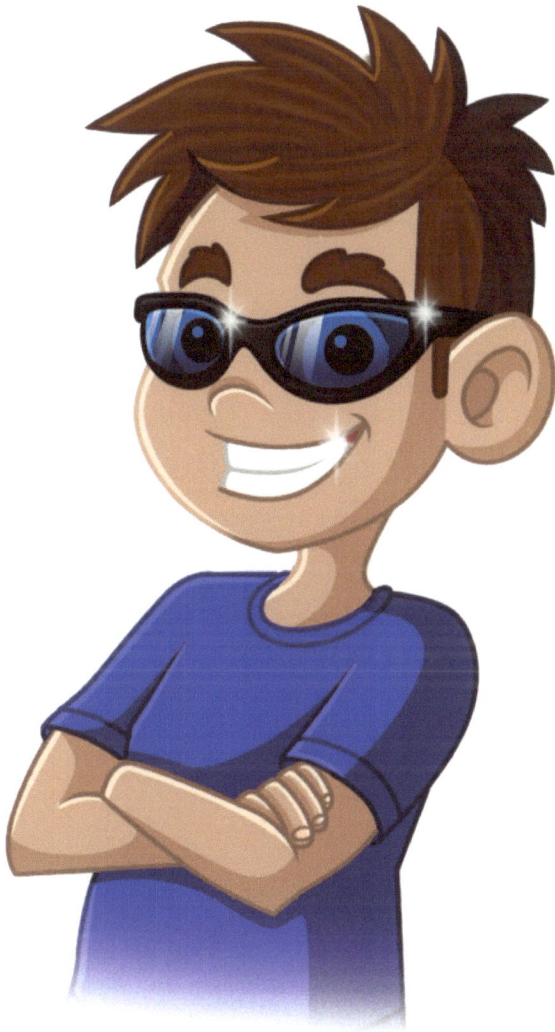

Now that I have everything together, it's time to load it all up and hit some <u>single track!</u>

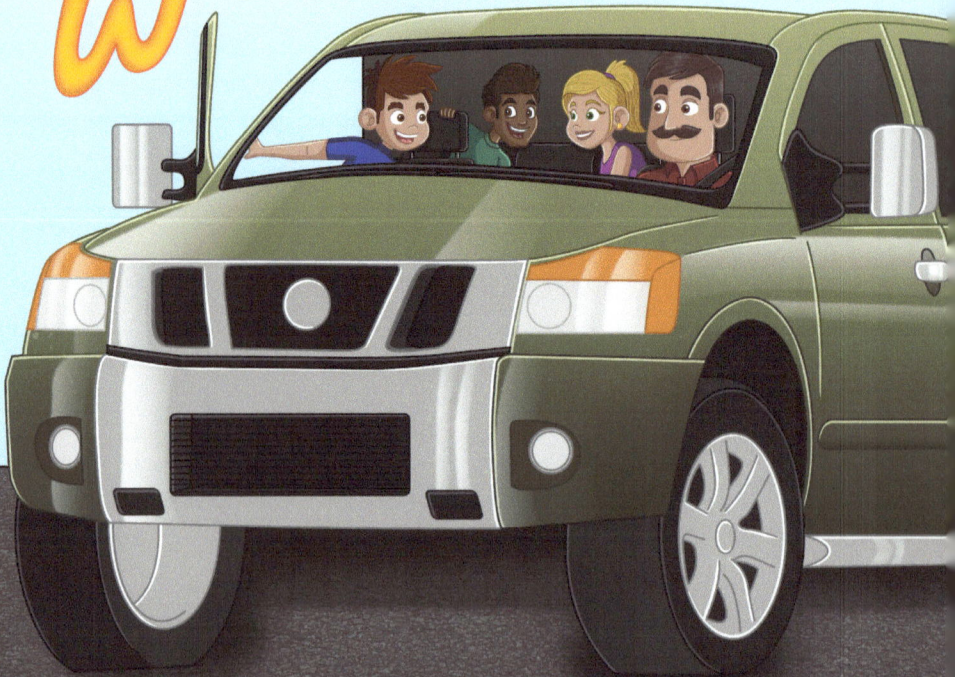

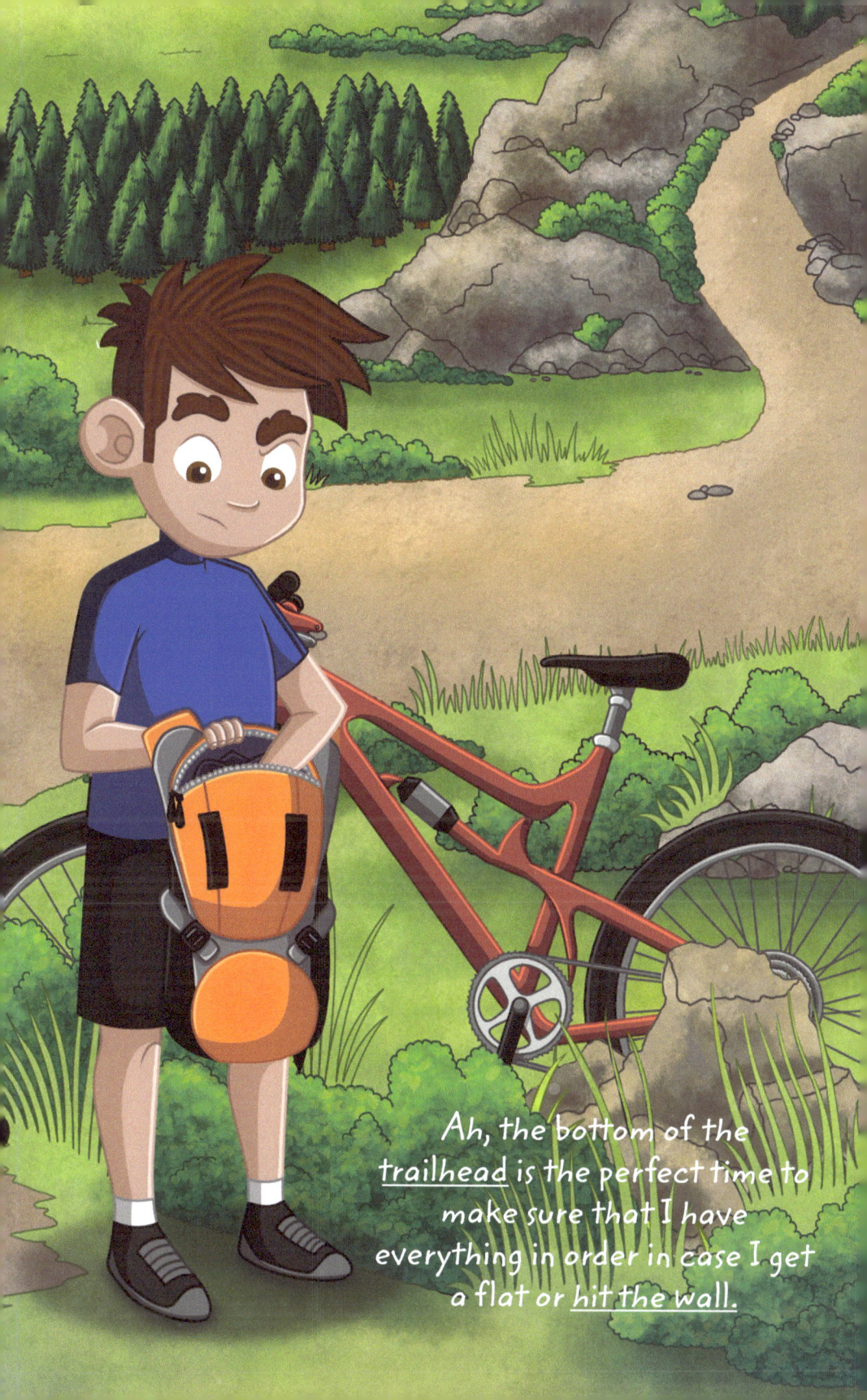

Ah, the bottom of the <u>trailhead</u> is the perfect time to make sure that I have everything in order in case I get a flat or <u>hit the wall</u>.

While everyone else is getting geared up to start, you and I have a chance to review some of the words we usually use when we bike.

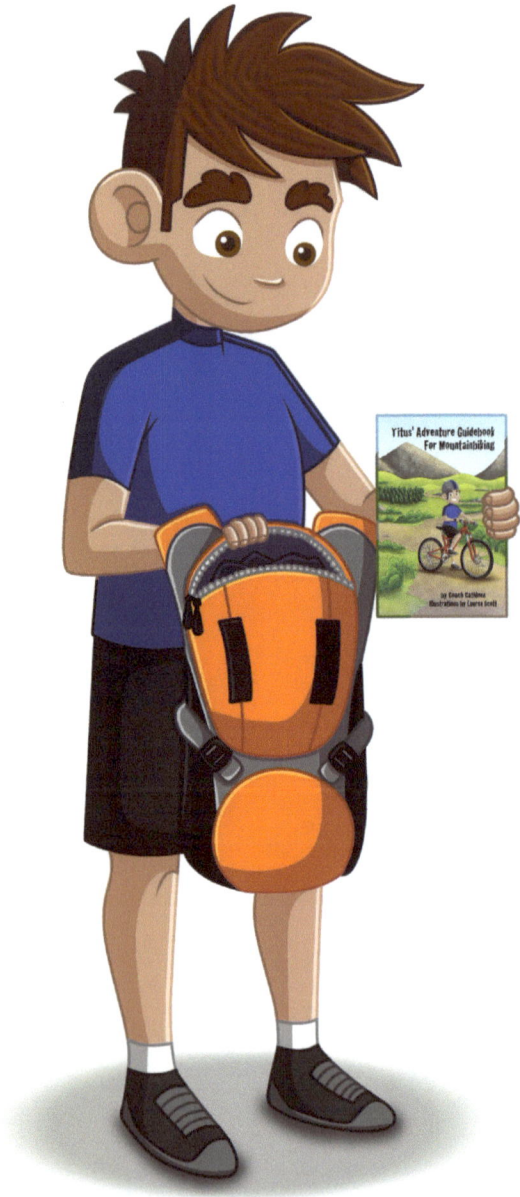

Common bike lingo:

Air: Space between the two tires and ground.

Bail: To quickly jump off the bike when in possible danger of crashing.

Bomb: Riding really fast downhill.

Bonk / Hit the wall: When you are overly tired or in dire need of fuel.

Death March: A long endurance ride usually involving a lot of uphill riding.

Double track: A trail wide enough for two people or bikes.

Endo: Flying over the handlebars and going end over end. This is commonly referred to as "going over the falls".

Fuel: Healthy snacks and water to boost your energy.

Granny gear: The lowest or easiest gear on your bike.

Single Track: A trail just wide enough for one bike.

Trailhead: The beginning of a mountain bike trail.

Okay, time to drop it in the <u>granny gear</u> and let the <u>death march</u> begin!

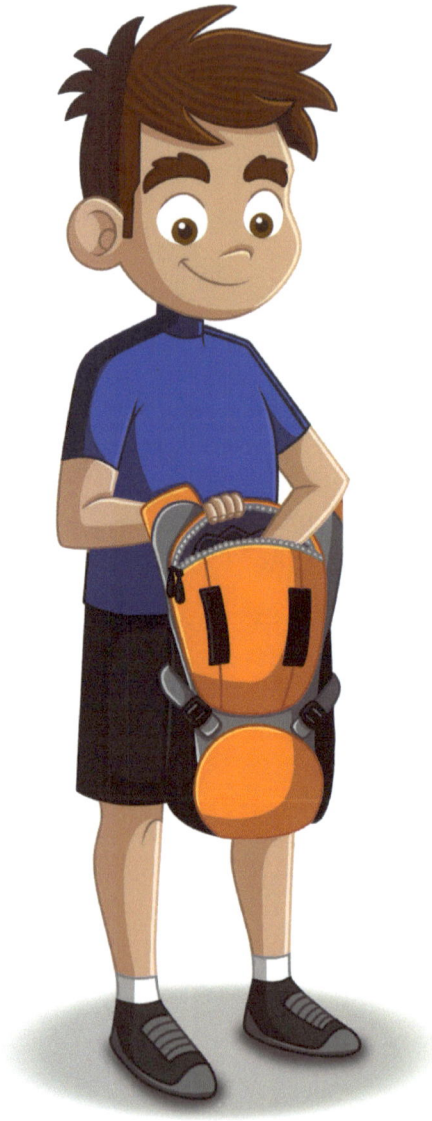

Remember to keep the rubber side down, stay safe, and have an awesome adventure!

See you on the trail!

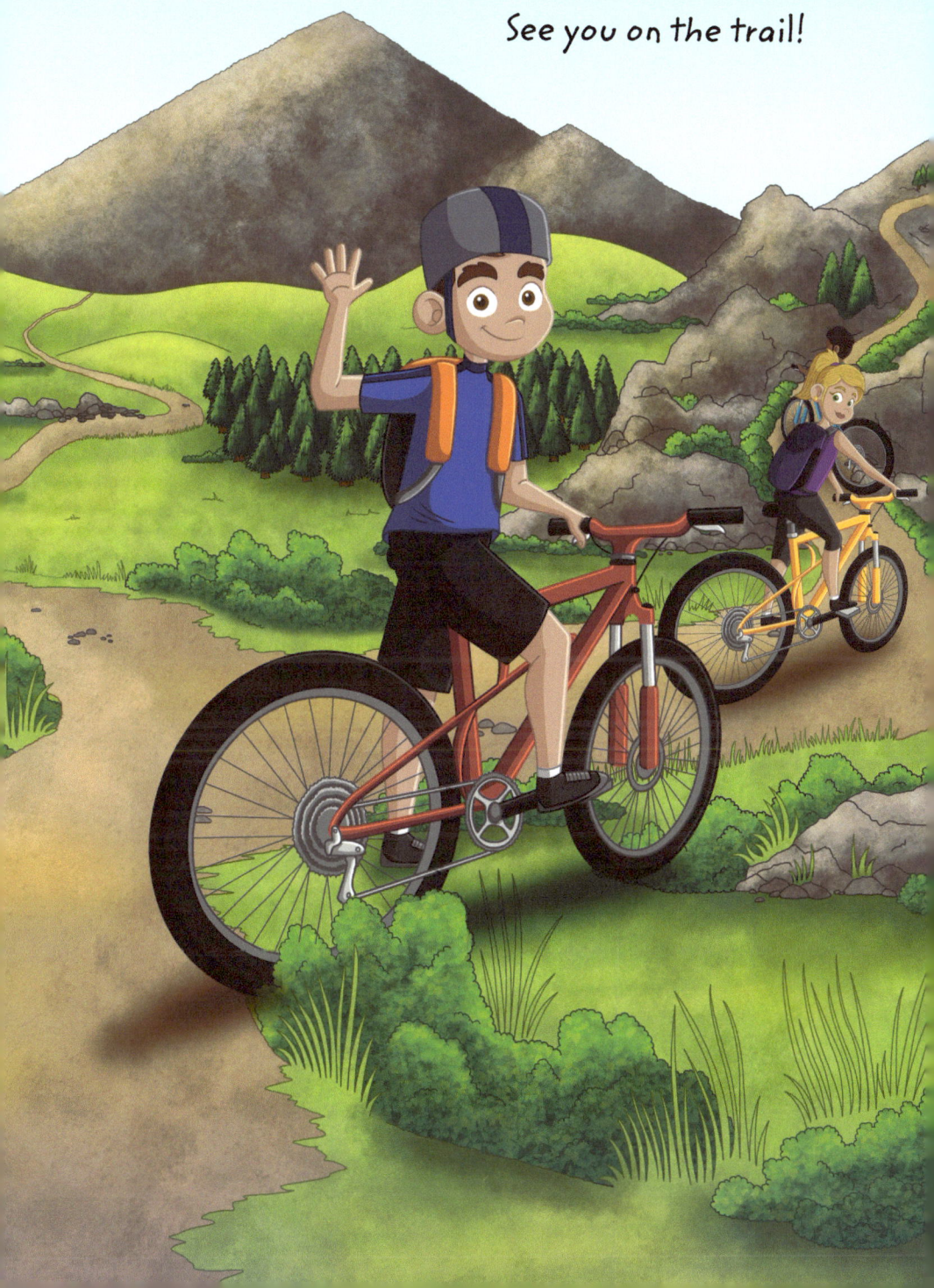

As a fitness trainer, Mother of two very active boys, and writer of the TAG series, Cathleen has to be pretty inventive in order to get out on her fat-tired adventures. Luckily, living in St. George, Utah provides lots of year round opportunities to get outside!

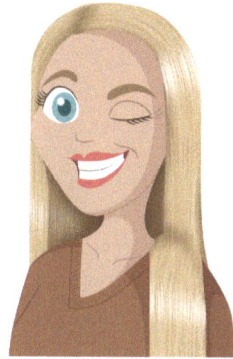

Lauren is an illustrator from London, UK. Loving everything art and animation related, she has been drawing since she was old enough to hold a pencil. When she isn't illustrating Lauren loves to travel, see new things, and have great adventures. www.lauren-scott.co.uk

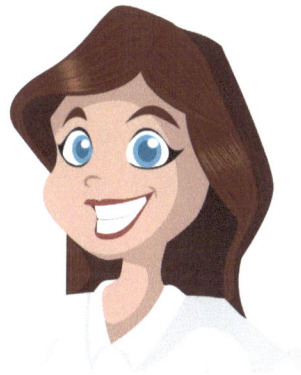

For latest updates on all the books in Titus' Adventure Guidebook (TAG) series, check us out online!

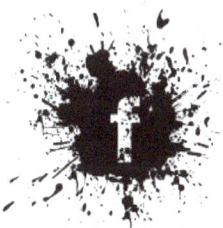

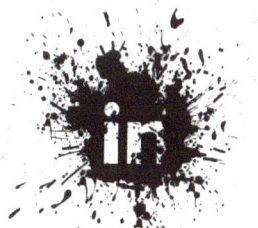

CCTfitness          Coach Cathleen          CoachCath

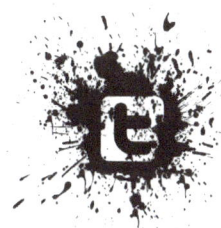

# Mountain Biking NOTES: